JUICING FOR DIABETES

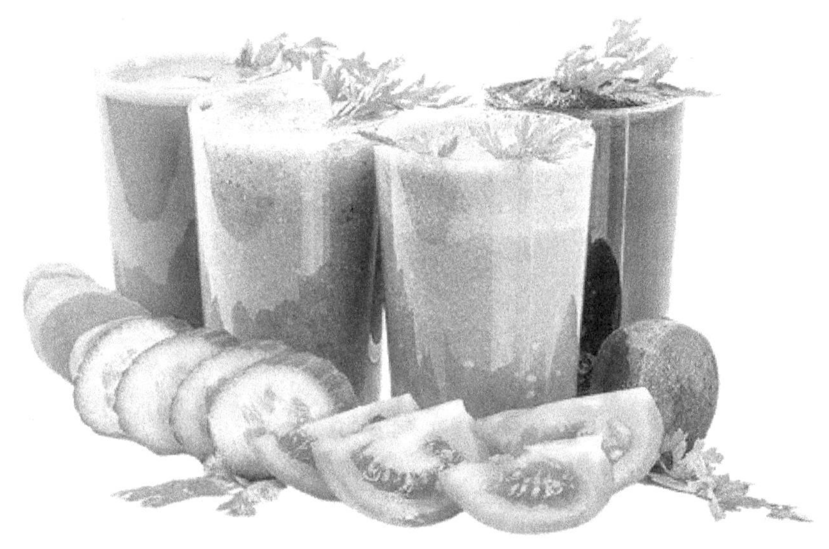

The Ultimate Guide To Lowering Your Blood Sugar And Improving Health

MIRIAM BROWN

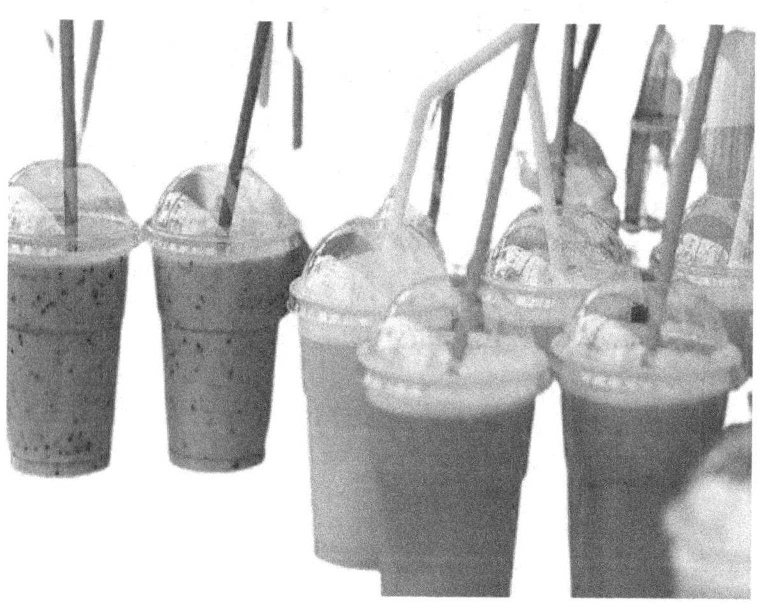

TABLE OF CONTENTS

INTRODUCTION

Greg was diagnosed with type 2 diabetes five years ago. At first, he struggled to control his blood sugar levels, despite taking medication and following a strict diet. Then he discovered the benefits of juicing.

Greg began incorporating fresh juices made from fruits and vegetables into his daily routine. He found that the nutrients in the juices helped to regulate his blood sugar levels and reduce inflammation in his body. Over time, he was able to reduce his medication and maintain healthy blood sugar levels with the help of juicing.

Despite his success, Greg faced skepticism from some members of his family and friends. They couldn't believe that juicing could have such a significant impact on his health. But Greg was determined to stick with it, and he even began sharing his knowledge with others who were struggling with diabetes.

One day, Greg's niece was diagnosed with type 2 diabetes. She was scared and overwhelmed, and didn't know where to turn for help. That's when Greg stepped in. He taught her about the benefits of juicing and helped her develop a routine that would work for her.

With Greg's guidance, his niece was able to reduce her medication and maintain healthy blood sugar levels. She was amazed at the difference that juicing had made in her life, and grateful for Greg's help and support.

In the end, Greg's success with juicing for diabetes inspired others to try it for themselves. He became a true champion of the practice, and continued to share his knowledge and experience with anyone who was willing to listen. Thanks to Greg's dedication and perseverance, many people with diabetes were able to improve their health and live happier, more fulfilling lives.

Millions of individuals throughout the world suffer with diabetes, a chronic disease. Managing diabetes requires a comprehensive approach that includes medication, lifestyle changes, and a healthy diet. Juicing is a popular method for getting important vitamins, minerals, and nutrients in a convenient and tasty way. For people with diabetes, juicing can be an effective way to regulate blood sugar levels, improve digestion, and boost overall health. In this book, we will explore the benefits of juicing for diabetes, including specific recipes that can help manage blood sugar levels and promote better health.

People with diabetes need to be mindful of their diet and nutrition because the condition affects the body's ability to produce or use insulin, a hormone that regulates blood sugar levels. High blood sugar levels can cause a range of health problems, including nerve damage, kidney damage, heart disease, and vision problems.

Therefore, it's important for people with diabetes to manage their blood sugar levels carefully by maintaining a healthy diet and getting regular exercise.

Juicing can be an effective way to supplement a healthy diet and provide essential nutrients to the body. By juicing fruits and vegetables, people with diabetes can consume a large amount of vitamins, minerals, and antioxidants in one convenient serving. Additionally, juicing can be a great way to incorporate more vegetables into the diet, which is especially important for people with diabetes who need to limit their intake of high-glycemic foods.

However, it's important to note that not all juicing recipes are suitable for people with diabetes. Some fruits and vegetables are high in sugar, which can cause blood sugar levels to spike. Therefore, it's important to choose recipes that are low in sugar and high in fiber, which can help regulate blood sugar levels and improve digestion.

Overall, juicing can be a beneficial addition to a diabetes management plan, but it's important to consult with a healthcare professional before making any significant changes to the diet or nutrition. In the following sections, we will explore the specific benefits of juicing for diabetes and provide recipes that are safe and effective for managing blood sugar levels.

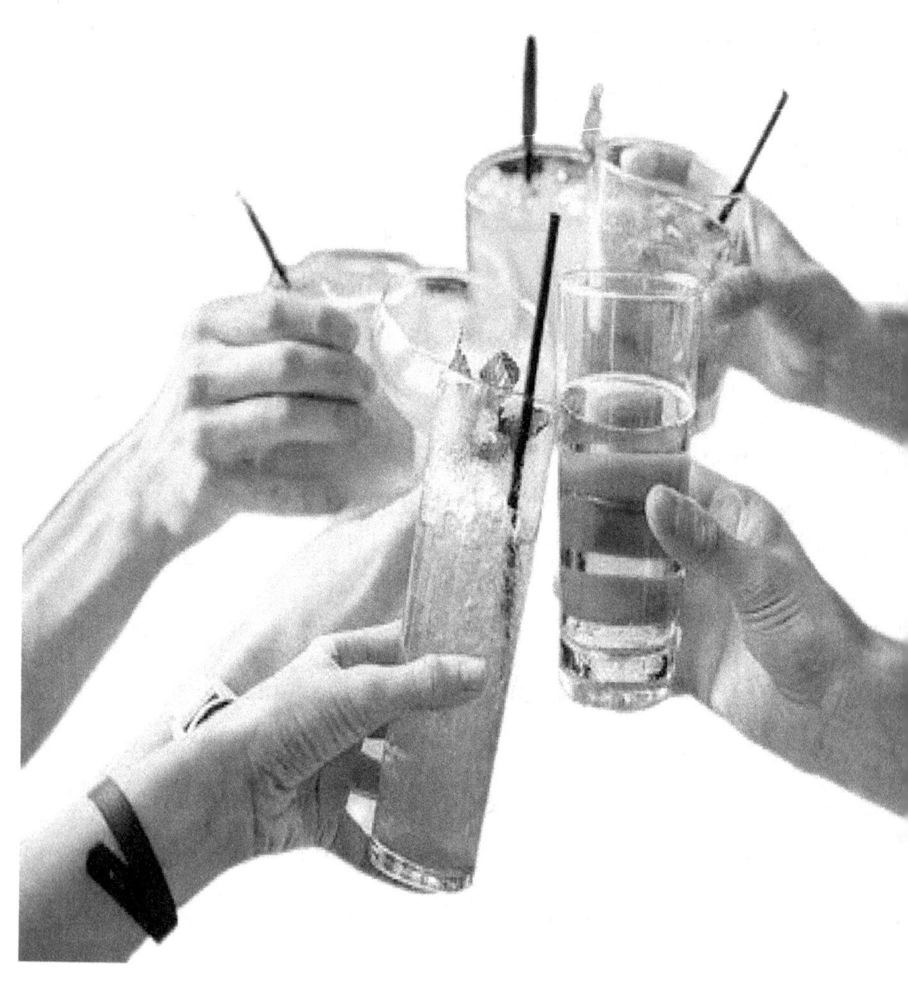

CHAPTER 1

SOME CONTEXT ON DIABETES AND HOW IT AFFECTS THE BODY

High blood glucose (sugar) levels are a defining feature of the chronic medical condition diabetes. Glucose is the main source of energy for the body's cells, and insulin, a hormone produced by the pancreas, helps to regulate the amount of glucose in the bloodstream.

Diabetes comes in two basic varieties: type 1 and type 2.Type 1 diabetes occurs when the body's immune system attacks and destroys the cells in the pancreas that produce insulin. Type 2 diabetes occurs when the body becomes resistant to insulin or doesn't produce enough insulin to maintain normal blood sugar levels.

Both types of diabetes can lead to high levels of glucose in the blood, which can cause a variety of health problems over time. Among the frequent consequences of diabetes are:

Diabetes can raise your chance of having a heart attack, a stroke, and other cardiovascular issues.

Nerve damage:

High blood sugar levels can damage the nerves throughout the body, leading to a variety of signs and symptoms such discomfort, tingling, and numbness.

Kidney damage:

Diabetes can damage the blood vessels in the kidneys, leading to kidney disease and eventually kidney failure.

Eye damage:

High blood sugar levels can damage the blood vessels in the eyes, leading to vision problems and, in severe cases, blindness.

Foot damage:

Nerve damage and poor circulation caused by diabetes can lead to foot problems, including infections, ulcers, and in severe cases, amputation.

Managing diabetes involves monitoring blood sugar levels, taking insulin or other medications as prescribed, making dietary changes, and engaging in regular physical activity. With proper management, many people with diabetes can live healthy, active lives and reduce their risk of complications.

However, if diabetes is left unmanaged, it can lead to serious and life-threatening complications. Therefore, it is crucial for individuals with diabetes to work closely with their healthcare team to develop a personalized treatment plan that meets their unique needs and lifestyle.

In addition to managing blood sugar levels, people with diabetes may need to make other lifestyle changes to reduce their risk of complications. This may include quitting smoking, maintaining a healthy weight, eating a balanced diet, and engaging in regular physical activity.

It is also important for people with diabetes to monitor their overall health and seek medical attention if they experience any unusual symptoms or changes in their health status. Regular check-ups with healthcare providers can help to identify and address any potential problems before they become more serious.

In summary, diabetes is a chronic medical condition that can have a significant impact on the body if left unmanaged. However, with proper treatment and lifestyle modifications, many people with diabetes can lead healthy, active lives and reduce their risk of complications.

TYPE 1 DIABETES AND HOW IT DIFFERS FROM TYPE 2 DIABETES.

Type 1 diabetes, also known as insulin-dependent diabetes or juvenile diabetes, is a chronic condition in which the body's immune system attacks and destroys insulin-producing cells in the pancreas .The hormone insulin regulates the blood's level of glucose (sugar). Without insulin, the body cannot properly use or store glucose, which can lead to high blood sugar levels and a variety of complications.

Despite the fact that it may occur at any age, type 1 diabetes is commonly discovered in children and young adults. Symptoms of type 1 diabetes can include increased thirst and urination, extreme hunger, weight loss, fatigue, blurred vision, and frequent infections. Treatment typically involves regular insulin injections or the use of an insulin pump, along with monitoring blood sugar levels and following a healthy diet and exercise plan.

If left untreated, type 1 diabetes can lead to serious complications, such as diabetic ketoacidosis (DKA), which is a life-threatening condition that occurs when the body breaks down fat instead of glucose for energy. Other complications can include nerve damage, kidney damage, eye problems, and cardiovascular disease.

Type 1 diabetes is thought to have a hereditary and environmental component, while its specific origin is unknown. There is no cure for type 1 diabetes, but with proper treatment and management, people with this condition can lead healthy, active lives.

It's important for people with type 1 diabetes to work closely with their healthcare team to manage their condition and prevent complications. This may involve monitoring blood sugar levels regularly, adjusting insulin doses as needed, following a healthy diet and exercise plan, and getting regular check-ups and screenings. Additionally, it's important for family members, friends, and coworkers to be aware of the signs and symptoms of type 1 diabetes, so that they can provide support and help in an emergency situation.

Type 1 diabetes and type 2 diabetes are two different conditions with distinct causes and treatment approaches.

Type 1 diabetes is an autoimmune disorder in which the body's immune system attacks and destroys the insulin-producing cells (beta cells) in the pancreas. As a result, people with type 1 diabetes do not produce enough insulin to regulate their blood sugar levels. Type 1 diabetes typically develops during childhood or adolescence, although it can also develop in adulthood.

On the other hand, type 2 diabetes is a metabolic disorder that develops when the body becomes resistant to insulin or does not produce enough insulin to maintain normal blood sugar levels. Obesity, inactivity, and poor diet are common lifestyle factors linked to type 2 diabetes. Type 2 diabetes typically develops in adulthood, although it can also develop in childhood or adolescence.

The symptoms of type 1 and type 2 diabetes can be similar, including increased thirst and urination, fatigue, and blurred vision. However, there are some differences in the symptoms that may help to distinguish between the two types. For example, people with type 1 diabetes often experience rapid weight loss, while people with type 2 diabetes may have a more gradual onset of symptoms.

The treatment of type 1 diabetes usually involves insulin therapy, which may be delivered through injections or an insulin pump. People with type 1 diabetes must carefully monitor their blood sugar levels and adjust their insulin doses accordingly to avoid complications such as diabetic ketoacidosis. In contrast, the treatment of type 2 diabetes may involve lifestyle changes such as weight loss, exercise, and diet modifications, as well as medications such as metformin, insulin, or other blood sugar-lowering drugs.

Overall, while both type 1 and type 2 diabetes affect the body's ability to regulate blood sugar levels, they differ in their underlying causes, age of onset, and treatment approaches.

In addition, there are some other differences between type 1 and type 2 diabetes. For instance, type 1 diabetes is much less common than type 2 diabetes, accounting for only about 5-10% of all diabetes cases. Type 2 diabetes is much more prevalent, affecting about 90-95% of people with diabetes.

Another difference is that people with type 1 diabetes are at higher risk for developing certain complications, such as diabetic ketoacidosis, which can be life-threatening if left untreated. People with type 2 diabetes may be more likely to develop other complications such as heart disease, stroke, and kidney damage.

It's important for people with both types of diabetes to carefully manage their condition in order to avoid complications and maintain good health. This may involve making lifestyle changes, taking medications as prescribed, monitoring blood sugar levels regularly, and working closely with a healthcare team to develop a personalized treatment plan.

In summary, while type 1 and type 2 diabetes share some similarities in terms of symptoms and complications, they are distinct conditions with different causes and treatment approaches. Understanding these differences can help people with diabetes and their healthcare providers to make informed decisions about managing their condition.

CHARACTERISTICS OF TYPE 2 DIABETES AND HOW IT AFFECTS THE BODY.

Type 2 diabetes is a chronic metabolic disorder that affects how your body uses glucose (sugar) for energy. It is characterized by high levels of glucose in the blood due to the body's inability to produce or effectively use insulin, a hormone that helps regulate blood sugar levels.

The following are the key characteristics of type 2 diabetes:

Insulin resistance:

People with type 2 diabetes are resistant to the action of insulin, which means that their bodies are not able to use insulin properly to control blood sugar levels.

High blood sugar levels:

This occurs when the body is unable to use glucose effectively, leading to a buildup of glucose in the blood.

Increased thirst and urination:

Due to high blood sugar levels, the body tries to flush out excess glucose through urine, leading to increased urination and thirst.

Fatigue:

The cells in the body are not getting enough energy due to high blood sugar levels, leading to feelings of fatigue and weakness.

Slow healing:

High blood sugar levels can also slow down the body's ability to heal from injuries or infections.

Blurred vision:

High blood sugar levels can damage the blood vessels in the eyes, leading to blurred vision or even blindness.

Numbness or tingling in the hands or feet:

Over time, high blood sugar levels can damage the nerves in the body, leading to numbness or tingling sensations in the hands or feet.

Increased risk of other health problems:

People with type 2 diabetes have an increased risk of developing other health problems such as heart disease, stroke, kidney disease, and nerve damage.

Over time, high blood sugar levels can lead to damage in many organs of the body. For example, the risk of heart disease and stroke is increased due to the damage caused to blood vessels, as well as the higher levels of inflammation in the body. Kidney damage can also occur, leading to reduced kidney function and the need for dialysis or kidney transplant in severe cases. Nerve damage can cause pain, numbness, or tingling sensations in the hands and feet, and in some cases, it can lead to a loss of sensation or even amputation.

In order to avoid complications, type 2 diabetes must be managed continuously. The management of type 2 diabetes typically involves a combination of lifestyle modifications, such as regular exercise, healthy eating habits, and weight loss, as well as medication to help control blood sugar levels. Medications may include oral drugs that help the body use insulin more effectively, injectable drugs that stimulate insulin production, or insulin therapy itself. Regular monitoring of blood sugar levels is also necessary to ensure that the condition is well-managed and to prevent complications.

In conclusion, type 2 diabetes is a serious condition that affects many aspects of the body's functioning. However, with appropriate management and treatment, people with type 2 diabetes can live healthy and fulfilling lives. It is important to maintain a healthy lifestyle, take medications as prescribed, and work closely with healthcare professionals to manage the condition effectively.

OTHER FORMS OF DIABETES, THEIR CAUSES AND SYMPTOMS
GESTATIONAL DIABETES:

Gestational diabetes is a condition that affects pregnant women and is characterized by elevated blood glucose levels. It typically occurs during the second or third trimester and usually resolves after the baby is born. While it can have serious implications for both mother and baby, most women with gestational diabetes are able to manage it through dietary and lifestyle changes.

Hormonal changes that take place during pregnancy are what create gestational diabetes. As the placenta grows, it produces hormones that interfere with the body's ability to use insulin, the hormone that helps cells absorb sugar. This leads to a buildup of sugar in the blood, which can cause complications for both mother and baby.

Increased thirst, frequent urination, exhaustion, and impaired eyesight are all signs of gestational diabetes. Women with gestational diabetes also have an increased risk of developing preeclampsia, a condition characterized by high blood pressure during pregnancy.

Risk factors for gestational diabetes include obesity, a family history of diabetes, and having had gestational diabetes in a previous pregnancy. Women of certain ethnic backgrounds, such as African American, Hispanic, and Native American, are also at higher risk.

Diet and exercise are the main treatments for gestational diabetes. It's important to maintain a healthy diet that is low in simple carbohydrates and high in fiber. Exercise can help reduce blood glucose levels and may also help reduce the risk of developing complications. Insulin injections could be required in specific circumstances.If gestational diabetes is managed properly, the risks to both mother and baby are minimal. However, it's important to speak with a doctor about any concerns or questions. With the right treatment plan, most women with gestational diabetes are able to have a healthy pregnancy and delivery.

LADA:

LADA, or latent autoimmune diabetes of adults, is a condition in which the body's immune system attacks its own pancreatic cells that are responsible for producing insulin. As a result, the body is unable to produce or use insulin properly, leading to elevated blood sugar levels and eventual diabetes.

The symptoms of LADA can be similar to those of type 1 and type 2 diabetes, but the condition can be difficult to diagnose due to its slow onset. Common symptoms include increased thirst, frequent urination, fatigue, blurred vision, and weight loss. If left untreated, the condition can lead to serious complications such as heart disease, stroke, nerve damage, and kidney failure.

The cause of LADA is not well understood, but research suggests that genetics, environmental factors, and autoimmune disorders can play a role. It is also believed that LADA can be triggered by certain viruses and other infections.

The primary treatment for LADA is insulin, which can be taken orally or through injection. Other medications, such as metformin, may also be prescribed to help manage blood sugar levels. Additionally, lifestyle modifications such as healthy eating, regular exercise, and stress management can help to manage the symptoms of LADA.

Although LADA is a serious condition, it can be managed through proper treatment and lifestyle modifications. By recognizing the symptoms of LADA early, individuals can take steps to prevent long-term complications and maintain their quality of life.

MODY:

MODY, or Maturity Onset Diabetes of the Young, is a genetic form of diabetes that usually affects people before the age of 25. It is a type of diabetes that is caused by a mutation in one of the genes responsible for making insulin.

The symptoms of MODY can vary widely, but generally include frequent urination, increased thirst, increased appetite, and fatigue. If left untreated, it can lead to complications such as vision loss, nerve damage, kidney damage, and heart disease.

The causes of MODY are the same as those for Type 1 and Type 2 diabetes. These include heredity, genetic mutations, and environmental factors such as obesity, lack of exercise, and poor diet.

There is no cure for MODY, but it can be managed with lifestyle and medication. Lifestyle changes such as diet, exercise, and weight management can help keep blood sugar levels within a healthy range. Additionally, medications such as insulin and oral medications can help manage and control the disease.

Though MODY is a serious condition, it can be managed with the right treatment plan. It is important to work closely with a doctor or diabetes specialist to ensure that the best plan is in place to keep blood sugar levels in check and avoid complications.

SECONDARY DIABETES:

Secondary diabetes is a form of diabetes that is caused by another medical condition or from taking a certain type of medication. Common causes of secondary diabetes include Cushing's syndrome, pancreatic diseases, and certain medications.

The most common symptom of secondary diabetes is high blood sugar levels. Other symptoms include excessive thirst, frequent urination, and weight loss. If left untreated, secondary diabetes can lead to complications, such as nerve damage and kidney damage.

The primary cause of secondary diabetes is an underlying medical condition. Cushing's syndrome is an endocrine disorder that causes the body to produce too much cortisol, leading to high blood sugar levels. Pancreatic diseases, such as pancreatitis and pancreatic cancer, can also cause secondary diabetes. Certain medications, such as steroids and birth control pills, can also affect blood sugar levels.

Treatment for secondary diabetes typically involves managing the underlying medical condition or stopping the medication that is causing the problem. In some cases, a combination of lifestyle changes and medication may be necessary. Lifestyle changes include following a healthy diet, exercising regularly, and maintaining a healthy weight. Medications such as insulin or oral diabetes medications may be prescribed to help control blood sugar levels.

Secondary diabetes is a serious condition that can lead to complications if left untreated. If you suspect that you have secondary diabetes, it is important to seek medical help right away. Your doctor can help you determine the underlying cause and determine the best course of treatment.

TYPE 3 DIABETES:

Type 3 diabetes is a condition in which the pancreas does not produce enough of the hormone insulin. It is often referred to as adult-onset, or late-onset diabetes. Type 3 diabetes is much less common than types 1 and 2, and typically affects adults in their mid-50s and older.

The most common symptom of type 3 diabetes is frequent urination, as well as excessive thirst and hunger. Other symptoms may include weight loss, fatigue, blurred vision, slow healing of cuts and bruises, and numbness or tingling in the hands and feet.

The exact cause of type 3 diabetes is unknown, however it is believed to be related to lifestyle factors such as obesity and a lack of physical activity. Other risk factors may include age, family history of diabetes, and certain medical conditions.

There is no cure for type 3 diabetes, however it can be managed with a healthy lifestyle, including a balanced diet and regular exercise. Additionally, medications such as insulin and oral medications may be prescribed to help regulate blood sugar levels.

Additionally, regular visits with a healthcare provider can help manage any complications related to diabetes.

It is important for those with type 3 diabetes to practice healthy lifestyle choices, such as maintaining a healthy weight, eating a balanced diet and exercising regularly. Additionally, those with type 3 diabetes should monitor their blood sugar levels regularly, and follow their healthcare provider's instructions for managing their condition. By making these lifestyle changes, those with type 3 diabetes can lead a healthy, active life.

CAUSES OF DIABETES
GENETICS:

Genetics is one of the causes of diabetes. The genetic component of diabetes is complex and scientists are still trying to understand the exact mechanism. While the exact cause of diabetes is not yet known, there are certain genetic mutations and alterations that can increase the risk of developing the disorder.

One of the most common genetic factors in the development of diabetes is the HLA gene. This gene helps the body recognize and respond to foreign substances and is found on chromosome 6. A mutation in this gene has been linked to an increased risk of developing type 1 diabetes.

Another gene that is responsible for diabetes is the insulin gene. This gene helps the body produce insulin and is located on chromosome 11. Mutations in this gene can lead to a reduction in the amount of insulin produced by the body, making it difficult for the body to regulate glucose levels.

In addition to mutations in these two genes, other genetic factors can increase the risk of developing diabetes. These include mutations in genes involved in the production of glucose, the transport of glucose, and the storage of glucose.

The role of genetics in diabetes is complex and scientists are still trying to understand the exact mechanism. However, it is clear that genetics plays a role in the development of this disorder. Knowing your family history and being aware of the genetic risk factors can help you to better manage your health and reduce your risk of developing diabetes.

In addition to genetics, other factors such as lifestyle and environmental factors can increase the risk of diabetes. Eating a healthy diet, maintaining an active lifestyle, and managing stress can all help to reduce the risk of developing diabetes.

In conclusion, genetics is one of the causes of diabetes. Mutations in certain genes can increase the risk of developing diabetes. It is important to be aware of your family history and the genetic risk factors for diabetes. In addition, lifestyle and environmental factors can also increase the risk of developing this disorder. By managing these risk factors, you can reduce your risk of developing diabetes.

OBESITY:

Obesity is a major cause of diabetes, particularly type 2 diabetes. Obesity is defined as a having a body mass index (BMI) of 30 or higher. Overweight people are those with a BMI of 25 or higher. People with a BMI of 18.5 to 24.9 are considered to be of normal weight.

When someone is obese, the body has difficulty using insulin properly. This is known as insulin resistance. Insulin is a hormone produced by the pancreas which helps the body break down sugar into energy. When the body is resistant to insulin, sugar builds up in the bloodstream instead of being used as energy. This leads to diabetes.

Obesity occurs when the energy intake and expenditure is not balanced. People consume more calories than they burn, leading to an increase in body weight. This imbalance is often caused by an unhealthy diet, lack of physical activity, or both. While genetics can also play a role in obesity, diet and exercise are the main contributing factors.

Obese individuals are at greater risk of developing type 2 diabetes. This is due to the aforementioned insulin resistance, as well as the fact that obesity is associated with other risk factors for diabetes, such as high blood pressure, high cholesterol, and a sedentary lifestyle.

In addition, obesity can lead to an increase in visceral fat, which is fat that is stored around the abdominal organs. This type of fat is more dangerous than subcutaneous fat, which is the fat that is stored just under the skin. Visceral fat has been linked to an increased risk of type 2 diabetes as well as other health problems such as heart disease, stroke, and cancer.

Furthermore, obesity can cause chronic inflammation, which has been linked to an increased risk of type 2 diabetes. Chronic inflammation is the body's natural response to infection and injury. In obese individuals, however, inflammation is often caused by the body's attempt to fight off excess fat. This can lead to type 2 diabetes due to the body's inability to process sugar properly.

The good news is that losing weight can reduce the risk of developing type 2 diabetes. A weight loss of 5-10% can significantly reduce the risk, and even modest weight loss can have positive effects. Regular physical activity and a healthy, balanced diet are important for maintaining a healthy weight and reducing the risk of diabetes.

In conclusion, obesity is a major cause of type 2 diabetes. People with a BMI of 30 or higher are at an increased risk of developing the condition. Losing weight, exercising regularly, and eating a healthy diet can reduce the risk. It is important to take steps to maintain a healthy weight and reduce the risk of diabetes.

INSULIN RESISTANCE:

Insulin resistance is a condition in which the body's cells fail to respond to the hormone insulin, resulting in increased levels of glucose in the blood. It is a common cause of diabetes and is becoming increasingly prevalent in the population.

Insulin is a hormone produced by the pancreas that helps the body to regulate its blood sugar levels by allowing glucose to enter cells from the bloodstream. When the body is insulin resistant, the cells fail to respond to the insulin, meaning that glucose cannot enter the cells, leading to a buildup of glucose in the blood. This can cause levels of glucose to reach dangerously high levels, leading to the development of diabetes.

There are a number of factors that can increase the risk of developing insulin resistance, including being overweight or obese, having a family history of diabetes, and having high blood pressure, high cholesterol or a sedentary lifestyle. In addition, certain medications, such as glucocorticoids and thiazolidinediones, can increase the risk of insulin resistance.

The most common symptom of insulin resistance is elevated blood sugar levels. Other symptoms may include increased thirst, increased hunger, fatigue, blurred vision, and frequent urination. If left untreated, insulin resistance can lead to serious complications such as heart disease, stroke, and kidney disease.

In order to prevent the development of insulin resistance and diabetes, it is important to maintain a healthy lifestyle. This entails having a balanced diet, working out frequently, and keeping a healthy weight. It is also important to monitor your blood glucose levels regularly and to make sure that you are getting enough sleep.

If you are diagnosed with insulin resistance, your doctor may recommend lifestyle changes and/or medications to help manage your condition. These may include medications that help to improve insulin sensitivity, such as metformin, or medications that help to reduce blood glucose levels, such as sulfonylureas.

In conclusion, insulin resistance is a common cause of diabetes and is becoming increasingly prevalent in the population. It is important to maintain a healthy lifestyle and to monitor your blood glucose levels regularly in order to prevent the development of insulin resistance and diabetes. If you are diagnosed with insulin resistance, your doctor may recommend lifestyle changes and/or medications to help manage your condition.

AUTOIMMUNE RESPONSE:

Autoimmune response is one of the causes of diabetes, which is a condition when the body's immune system mistakenly attacks and destroys the cells in the pancreas that produce insulin. The body's blood sugar levels are regulated by the hormone insulin. If the body doesn't produce enough insulin, it can lead to high levels of glucose in the blood, which can cause serious health problems.

Autoimmune response is when the body's immune system mistakenly attacks its own cells, tissues, and organs. The body's immune system is supposed to protect the body from infections and other threats, but when it mistakenly attacks the body's own cells, it can cause serious health issues, such as diabetes.

With type 1 diabetes, the cells that make insulin in the pancreas are wrongly attacked and destroyed by the body's immune system. This can lead to a lack of insulin and high levels of glucose in the blood, which can cause serious health problems.

In type 2 diabetes, the body's immune system mistakenly attacks and destroys the cells that produce insulin, but this doesn't necessarily lead to a lack of insulin. In some cases, the body can still produce enough insulin

PANCREATIC DISEASE OR INJURY:

Pancreatic disease or injury is one of the main causes of diabetes, a condition in which the body's ability to produce or use insulin is impaired. Insulin is necessary for the body to be able to convert glucose, or sugar, into energy. Diabetes can be caused by a variety of factors, but pancreatic disease or injury is one of the most common causes.

Below the stomach sits an organ called the pancreas.It is responsible for producing hormones, such as insulin, that are necessary for the body to be able to process and use glucose. Pancreatic disease or injury can range from mild to severe, and any degree of damage can lead to diabetes. In some cases, the pancreas is completely destroyed and the body is unable to produce insulin at all. This is known as type 1 diabetes, and it requires lifelong insulin therapy.

Pancreatic disease or injury can be caused by a number of different factors. In some cases, it is caused by genetics, while in others it is caused by autoimmune disorders, such as celiac disease or cystic fibrosis. Viral or bacterial infections can also cause pancreatic damage, as can certain medications, such as steroids or chemotherapy drugs. In some cases, pancreatic disease or injury can be caused by trauma, such as a car accident or physical attack.

There are several symptoms of pancreatic disease or injury that can help diagnose diabetes. These include unexplained weight loss, increased thirst, frequent urination, fatigue, and blurred vision. If any of these symptoms are present, it is important to seek medical attention as soon as possible in order to diagnose and treat the condition.

Treatment for pancreatic disease or injury depends on the severity of the condition. In some cases, medications may be effective in controlling the symptoms and restoring insulin production. In more severe cases, surgery may be required to remove part or all of the pancreas. In some cases, an artificial pancreas may be implanted to replace the damaged pancreas.

Pancreatic disease or injury is one of the main causes of diabetes, a condition in which the body's ability to produce or use insulin is impaired. It is important to be aware of the symptoms of pancreatic disease or injury and seek medical attention as soon as possible in order to diagnose and treat the condition. Treatment options vary depending on the severity of the condition, but in many cases medications and/or surgery may be necessary in order to restore insulin production and control diabetes.

MEDICATIONS:

Medications, such as certain steroids and antipsychotics, can interfere with a person's ability to regulate blood sugar levels. Steroid medications, in particular, are known to cause an increase in blood glucose levels. Over time, this can lead to an increased risk of developing diabetes.

Antipsychotic medications can also interfere with the body's ability to regulate glucose levels. This is because these medications can affect the way the body produces or uses insulin. As a result, blood glucose levels can become elevated, leading to an increased risk of diabetes.

In addition to these two classes of medications, some other medications may also increase the risk of diabetes. These include certain hormones, such as those used to treat infertility and birth control pills. These medications can also interfere with the body's ability to regulate glucose levels, leading to an increased risk of diabetes.

Finally, certain medications used to treat high cholesterol, high blood pressure, and depression can also increase the risk of developing diabetes. These medications can interfere with the body's ability to properly regulate blood sugar levels, leading to an increased risk of diabetes.

It is important to note that these medications must be taken as directed in order to reduce the risk of developing diabetes. In most cases, these medications should only be taken if prescribed by a healthcare provider. It is also important to discuss any medications that may interfere with blood sugar regulation with the healthcare provider to ensure that the medications are being taken as safely and effectively as possible.

In conclusion, certain medications can increase the risk of developing diabetes. These medications include certain steroids, antipsychotics, hormones, high cholesterol medications, high blood pressure medications, and depression medications. Therefore, it is important to discuss any medications that may interfere with blood sugar regulation with a healthcare provider to ensure that the medications are being taken as safely and effectively as possible.

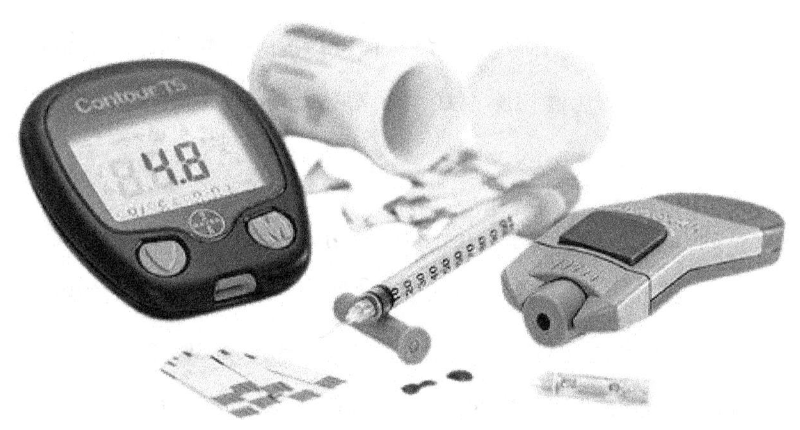

CHAPTER 2

UNDERSTANDING THE BASICS OF JUICING FOR DIABETES

Juicing for diabetes can be a great way to get the nutrients your body needs while controlling your blood sugar levels. Juicing allows you to control the amount of sugar and carbohydrates in your juice, making it easier to manage your diabetes. Juicing also gives you the opportunity to get nutrients from fruits and vegetables that you may not otherwise eat. In this book, we will explore the basics of juicing for diabetes, the benefits, and tips on how to get started.

First, let's look at the basics of juicing for diabetes. When juicing, it's important to keep in mind that it's best to avoid or limit high sugar fruits such as bananas, mangos, and pineapple. Instead, focus on lower sugar fruits such as apples, grapes, and citrus fruits. It's also important to avoid juices high in carbohydrates such as juice from carrots, beets, and other root vegetables.

The next step is to consider the type of juice you're making. If you're using a juicer, it's best to choose fresh fruits and vegetables that are in season. This way, you're getting the most nutrients from them. It's also important to use organic produce if possible.

Next, you'll want to think about the types of nutrients you're looking for in your juice. Most importantly, you'll want to make sure that you're getting enough vitamins and minerals. Vitamins A, C, and E are important for regulating blood sugar levels, and you'll want to make sure you're getting enough of these. Additionally, potassium and magnesium are important minerals for managing diabetes, and juicing is a great way to get more of these minerals in your diet.

Once you've got all the basics down, you'll want to start experimenting with different juice recipes. It's best to start with simple recipes and then gradually add more complex flavors and ingredients. For example, try adding a few tablespoons of flaxseed oil to your juice for an extra boost of omega-3 fatty acids. You can also add some fresh ginger or turmeric for an anti-inflammatory boost.

Juicing for diabetes can be a great way to get the nutrients your body needs while controlling your blood sugar levels. With a few simple tips and a bit of experimentation, you can create delicious, nutrient-packed juices that will help you manage your diabetes. So, get creative and start juicing today!

HOW DOES JUICING WORK?

Juicing is the process of extracting the liquid content from fruits and vegetables, leaving behind the pulp. The liquid that is extracted is commonly referred to as juice. The juice contains most of the vitamins, minerals, and other nutrients found in the fruits and vegetables, making it a popular way to consume a large amount of nutrients in one drink.

The process of juicing typically involves using a juicer, which grinds and squeezes the fruits and vegetables to separate the juice from the pulp. Some juicers use centrifugal force to extract the juice, while others use a hydraulic press.

Juicing can be done with a variety of fruits and vegetables, and many people enjoy creating their own unique blends. Popular ingredients for juicing include apples, carrots, celery, spinach, kale, beets, ginger, and citrus fruits.

Juicing is believed to have a number of health benefits, including providing a quick and convenient way to consume a large amount of vitamins and minerals, boosting energy levels, improving digestion, and supporting the immune system. However, it is important to note that juicing can also be high in sugar and low in fiber, so it should be consumed in moderation and as part of a balanced diet.

TYPES OF JUICING:
 Cold-pressed juicing:

Cold-pressed juicing is a type of juicing where the fruit and vegetables are crushed and then pressed to extract the maximum amount of juice, without using heat. This method preserves all the natural nutrients and enzymes in the juice, and results in a higher quality and nutrient-dense juice.

Centrifugal juicing:

Centrifugal juicing is the most common type of juicing. It involves using a high-speed spinning blade to extract juice from the fruits and vegetables. This method is fast and efficient, but it also produces a lot of heat and oxidation, which can degrade the quality of the juice and reduce the amount of vitamins and minerals.

Masticating juicing:

Masticating juicing is a type of juicing that uses a slower, more gentle approach. It uses a single auger or gear to crush and press the fruits and vegetables, resulting in a higher quality juice with more nutrients and enzymes.

Tribest juicing:

Tribest juicing is a type of juicing that uses a combination of masticating and centrifugal juicing. The Tribest juicer has both a masticating and centrifugal juicer built into one machine, making it a very versatile option for juicing.

High-pressure juicing:

High-pressure juicing is a type of juicing that uses a high-pressure process to extract juice from the fruit and vegetables. This method preserves the maximum amount of vitamins, minerals, and enzymes in the juice, resulting in a higher quality and nutrient-dense juice.

NUTRITIONAL BENEFITS OF JUICING

- Juicing can increase the amount of vitamins, minerals and other important nutrients that you get from your diet. By juicing, you can consume more fruits and vegetables in liquid form that would otherwise be hard to eat.

- Juicing can help improve digestion and absorption of essential nutrients from food. It can also help to detoxify the body, as the nutrients in the juice can help to flush out toxins.

- It can help to boost your energy levels due to the high vitamin and mineral content.

- Juicing can help to support a healthy immune system. The antioxidants and other nutrients in the juice can help to fight off infections and diseases.

- It can help to promote healthy weight loss. The nutrients in the juice can help to boost metabolism and burn fat more efficiently.

- Juicing can help to reduce inflammation in the body. The nutrients in the juice can help to reduce inflammation and pain.

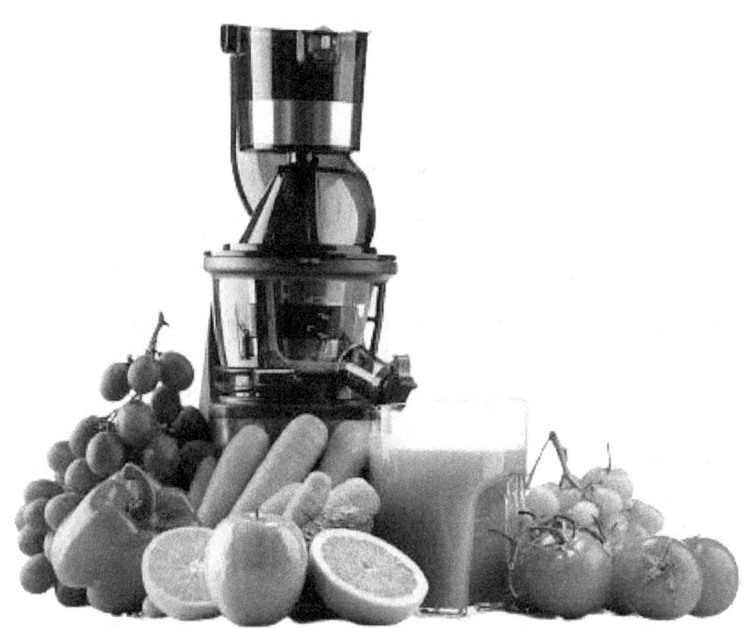

CHAPTER 3

JUICING RECIPES FOR DIABETES

Green Juice

This green juice recipe is packed with nutrients and antioxidants that can help regulate blood sugar levels and improve diabetes symptoms. The combination of spinach, cucumber, green apple, lemon and spirulina is full of vitamins and minerals that can help support healthy blood sugar levels. The addition of ground cinnamon and raw honey can help to sweeten the juice without adding refined sugar. Enjoy this green juice to support healthy blood sugar levels and to get a nutritious boost.

Ingredients:

-1 cup of spinach

-1 cucumber

-1/2 green apple

-1/4 lemon

-1 teaspoon of spirulina

-1/4 teaspoon of ground cinnamon

-1/4 teaspoon of raw honey

Instructions:

1. Wash the spinach, cucumber and green apple.

2. Cut the cucumber and apple into small pieces.

3. Add the spinach, cucumber, apple and lemon to a blender or food processor and blend until smooth.

4. Pour the juice into a glass and add the spirulina, cinnamon and honey.

5. Stir the ingredients together and enjoy.

Benefits of the Ingredients:

Cucumber: Cucumbers are a good source of vitamin K, which is important for bone health, and they also contain antioxidants that may help to reduce inflammation in the body.

Celery: Celery is a low-calorie vegetable that is rich in fiber and vitamin K. It also contains antioxidants that may help to reduce inflammation and improve heart health.

Green Apple: Green apples are a good source of vitamin C, which is important for immune health, and they also contain antioxidants that may help to reduce the risk of chronic diseases.

Lemon: Lemons are a good source of vitamin C and also contain antioxidants that may help to reduce inflammation and improve digestive health.

Ginger: Ginger has anti-inflammatory properties and may help to reduce nausea and improve digestion.

Spinach: An abundant source of vitamins A, C, and K, iron, folate, and other nutrients, spinach is a vegetable. It also contains antioxidants that may help to reduce inflammation and improve heart health.

Kale: Kale is another nutrient-dense vegetable that is high in vitamins A, C, and K, as well as calcium and iron. It also contains antioxidants that may help to reduce inflammation and improve heart health.

Parsley: Parsley is a good source of vitamin K, which is important for bone health, and also contains antioxidants that may help to reduce inflammation and improve digestion.

Mint: Mint has a refreshing flavor and may help to soothe digestive issues, such as indigestion and bloating.

Citrus Juice

Citrus juice is an excellent choice for diabetics as it is packed with vitamin C and antioxidants. Here is a delicious and healthy citrus juice recipe for diabetics:

Ingredients:

- 1 orange

- 1 grapefruit

- 2 lemons

- 1/2 cup of pineapple juice

- 1 teaspoon of honey

Instructions:

1. Peel and juice the orange, grapefruit, and lemons.

2. Add the pineapple juice and honey.

3. Mix all the ingredients together.

4. Pour into a glass and enjoy!

Benefits of each ingredient:

Oranges

Oranges are a great source of vitamin C, a powerful antioxidant that helps protect your cells from damage. Vitamin C also helps support your immune system and can help reduce inflammation in the body.

Grapefruits

Grapefruits are also high in vitamin C and contain other antioxidants, such as beta-carotene and lycopene. They may help lower cholesterol levels and promote weight loss.

Lemon

Lemons are a good source of vitamin C and also contain other antioxidants, such as flavonoids. Lemon juice may help improve digestion, boost immunity, and support healthy skin.

Lime

Limes are another good source of vitamin C and contain other antioxidants, such as flavonoids and limonoids. Lime juice may help improve digestion, reduce inflammation, and support healthy skin and hair.

Carrot Juice

Carrot juice is an incredibly healthy and nourishing drink that can be beneficial for people with diabetes. Rich in vitamins, minerals, and antioxidants, carrot juice can help to stabilize blood sugar levels and reduce the risk of complications associated with diabetes.

Ingredients:

-4-5 carrots

-1 teaspoon of ground ginger

-1 teaspoon of ground cinnamon

-1 tablespoon of honey

Instructions:

1. Wash and peel the carrots.

2. Cut the carrots into small pieces and add them to a blender.

3. Add the ground ginger, cinnamon and honey to the blender.

4. Blend the ingredients on a high speed until the mixture is smooth.

5. Strain the juice through a fine mesh sieve and discard the pulp.

6.Put the juice in a glass, then sip it.

Benefits:

Carrot juice is a great source of dietary fiber, which helps to slow down the absorption of sugar into the bloodstream, thus preventing spikes in blood sugar levels. The vitamins and minerals in carrot juice can also help to reduce inflammation and improve insulin sensitivity, which can help to reduce the risk of diabetes complications.

Ginger Lemonade

Ingredidents:

- 2-3 lemons,
- 2 inches fresh ginger root,
- 2 tablespoons honey,
- 2 cups cold water.

Instruction:

1. After peeling, slice the ginger root into small pieces.
2. Squeeze the lemon juice into a blender and add the ginger pieces. Mix everything together until a pastey consistency forms.
3. Add honey, cold water and mix until combined. Serve chilled.

Apple Beet Juice

1 apple

1 beet,

2 stalks celery

1/2 lemon.

Wash, peel and chop the apple and beet into small pieces. Add the celery stalks and lemon juice to a blender and blend until smooth. Juice may now be served by pouring it into a glass.

3. Carrot Orange Juice - 2 carrots, 1 orange, 1/2 teaspoon ground ginger. Carrots should be washed, peeled, and cut into small pieces. Slice the orange thinly after being peeled. Add the carrot and orange pieces to a blender and blend until smooth. Mix well after adding the ground ginger. Serve cold.

4. Mango Cucumber Juice - 1 mango, 1 cucumber, 1/2 teaspoon ground turmeric. Peel, pit and chop the mango into small pieces. The cucumber should be peeled and finely chopped. Add the mango and cucumber pieces to a blender and blend until smooth. Add the ground turmeric and mix until combined. Serve chilled.

5. Celery Pineapple Juice - 2 stalks celery, 1/2 pineapple, 1/2 teaspoon ground cinnamon. Wash, then cut the celery into little pieces. Peel, core and chop the pineapple into small pieces. Add the celery and pineapple pieces to a blender and blend until smooth. Add the ground cinnamon and mix until combined. Serve chilled.

6. Pear Kale Juice - 1 pear, 2 handfuls kale, 1/2 teaspoon ground nutmeg. Wash and chop the pear into small pieces. The kale should be washed and finely chopped. Add the pear and kale pieces to a blender and blend until smooth. Add the ground nutmeg and mix until combined. Serve chilled.

7. Watermelon Coconut Juice - 1 cup watermelon, 3/4 cup coconut water, 1/2 teaspoon ground cardamom. Peel, de-seed and chop the watermelon into small pieces. Add the watermelon pieces and

coconut water to a blender and blend until smooth. Add the ground cardamom and mix until combined. Serve chilled.

8. Kiwi Spinach Juice - 2 kiwis, 2 handfuls spinach, 1/2 teaspoon ground ginger. The kiwis should be peeled and chopped into little pieces. The spinach should be cleaned and finely chopped. Add the kiwi and spinach pieces to a blender and blend until smooth. Blend in the ground ginger after adding it. Serve chilled.

9. Grapefruit Mint Juice - 1 grapefruit, 10 mint leaves, 1/2 teaspoon ground cumin. Peel and cut the grapefruit into small pieces. The mint leaves should be washed and minced. Add the grapefruit and mint pieces to a blender and blend until smooth. Add the ground cumin and mix until combined. Serve chilled.

10. Plum Radish Juice - 2 plums, 3 radishes, 1/2 teaspoon ground coriander. Wash, de-seed and chop the plums into small pieces. Wash, peel and chop the radishes into small pieces. Add the plum and radish pieces to a blender and blend until smooth. Add the ground coriander and mix until combined. Serve chilled.

1. Coconut Broccoli Juice – 1/4 cup of coconut water, 1/4 cup of coconut milk, 1 cup of broccoli florets, 1/4 cup of spinach leaves,

1/2 teaspoon of lemon juice. Preparation: combine all the ingredients in a blender and process until completely smooth.

2. Blueberry Carrot Juice – 1/2 cup of blueberries, 1 large carrot, 1/2 cup of apple juice, 1/4 cup of spinach leaves, 1/4 teaspoon of turmeric powder. Preparation: Put all the ingredients in a blender and process until completely smooth.

3. Cucumber Beet Juice – 1 cucumber, 1/2 beet, 1/2 inch piece of ginger, 1/2 cup of spinach leaves, 1/2 cup of apple juice. Preparation: Peel and chop the cucumber and beet and place in a blender. Add the ginger, spinach leaves and apple juice and blend until smooth.

4. Peach Coconut Juice – 1 large peach, 1/4 cup of coconut milk, 1/4 cup of coconut water, 1/4 teaspoon of turmeric powder, 1/4 teaspoon of cinnamon powder. Preparation: Peel and chop the peach and place in a blender. Add the coconut milk, coconut water, turmeric powder and cinnamon powder and blend until smooth.

5. Grape Tomato Juice – 1 cup of grape tomatoes, 1/2 cup of orange juice, 1/4 cup of spinach leaves, 1/4 teaspoon of cumin powder. Preparation: combine all the ingredients in a blender and process until completely smooth.

6. Orange Spinach Juice – 2 oranges, 1 cup of spinach leaves, 1/4 cup of apple juice, 1/4 teaspoon of ginger powder. Preparation: Peel and chop the oranges and place in a blender. Add the spinach leaves, apple juice and ginger powder and blend until smooth.

7. Plum Celery Juice – 2 plums, 1 stalk of celery, 1/2 cup of spinach leaves, 1/4 cup of orange juice. Preparation: Peel and chop the plums and place in a blender. Add the celery, spinach leaves and orange juice and blend until smooth.

8. Lemon Kale Juice – 1 lemon, 1 cup of kale leaves, 1/2 cup of spinach leaves, 1/4 cup of apple juice. Preparation: Peel and chop the lemon and place in a blender. Add the kale leaves, spinach leaves and apple juice and blend until smooth.

9. Mango Lettuce Juice – 1 mango, 1/2 head of lettuce, 1/4 cup of coconut milk, 1/4 cup of coconut water. Preparation: Peel and chop the mango and place in a blender. Add the lettuce, coconut milk and coconut water and blend until smooth.

10. Papaya Parsley Juice – 1/2 papaya, 1/4 cup of parsley leaves, 1/2 cup of orange juice, 1/4 teaspoon of ginger powder. Preparation: Peel and chop the papaya and place in a blender. Add the parsley leaves, orange juice and ginger powder and blend until smooth.

1. Avocado Tomato Juice

Ingredients:

- 1 Avocado

- 2 Tomatoes

- 1/4 Cup Water

Preparation:

- Peel and cube the avocado.

- Cut the tomatoes into cubes.

- Place the avocado and tomato cubes into a blender and blend until smooth.

- Blend after adding the water for a further minute.

- Strain the juice and serve.

2. Cantaloupe Cucumber Juice

Ingredients:

- 1/2 Cantaloupe

- 1/2 Cucumber

- 1/4 Cup Water

Preparation:

- Peel and cube the cantaloupe.

- Peel and cube the cucumber.

- Place the cantaloupe and cucumber cubes into a blender and blend until smooth.

- Blend after adding the water for a further minute.

- Strain the juice and serve.

3. Apple Radish Juice

Ingredients:

- 1 Apple

- 2 Radishes

- 1/4 Cup Water

Preparation:

- Peel and core the apple.

- Cut the radishes into cubes.

- Place the apple and radish cubes into a blender and blend until smooth.

Blend after adding the water for a further minute.

- Strain the juice and serve.

4. Watermelon Grape Juice

Ingredients:

- 1/2 Watermelon

- 1/2 Cup Grapes

- 1/4 Cup Water

Preparation:

- Peel and cube the watermelon.

- Place the watermelon and grapes into a blender and blend until smooth.

Blend after adding the water for a further minute.

- Strain the juice and serve.

5. Pineapple Celery Juice

Ingredients:

- 1/2 Pineapple

- 2 Celery Stalks

- 1/4 Cup Water

Preparation:

- Peel and cube the pineapple.

- Cut the celery stalks into cubes.

- Place the pineapple and celery cubes into a blender and blend until smooth.

- Blend after adding the water for a further minute.

- Strain the juice and serve.

1. Peach Mint Juice - Ingredients: 2 peaches, 1 cup mint leaves, 1 cup of water. Preparation Technique: Peel and chop the peaches. Place the chopped peaches, mint leaves, and water in a blender. Blend until smooth. Serve the mixture after straining it through a sieve.

2. Carrot Parsley Juice - Ingredients: 3 carrots, 1 cup parsley leaves, 1 cup of water. Preparation Technique: Peel and chop the carrots. Place the chopped carrots, parsley leaves, and water in a blender. Blend until smooth. Serve the mixture after straining it through a sieve.

3. Kiwi Beet Juice - Ingredients: 2 kiwis, 1 beet, 1 cup of water. Preparation Technique: Peel and chop the kiwis. Peel and grate the beet. Place the chopped kiwis, grated beet, and water in a blender.

Blend until smooth. Serve the mixture after straining it through a sieve.

4. Lemon Broccoli Juice - Ingredients: 2 lemons, 2 cups broccoli florets, 1 cup of water. Preparation Technique: Peel and chop the lemons. Place the chopped lemons, broccoli florets, and water in a blender. Blend until smooth. Serve the mixture after straining it through a sieve.

5. Avocado Lettuce Juice - Ingredients: 1 avocado, 2 cups lettuce leaves, 1 cup of water. Preparation Technique: Peel and pit the avocado. Place the avocado, lettuce leaves, and water in a blender. Blend until smooth. Serve the mixture after straining it through a sieve.

6. Coconut Spinach Juice - Ingredients: 1 cup coconut milk, 2 cups spinach leaves, 1 cup of water. Preparation Technique: Place the coconut milk, spinach leaves, and water in a blender. Blend until smooth. Serve the mixture after straining it through a sieve.

7. Blueberry Radish Juice - Ingredients: 1 cup blueberries, 2 radishes, 1 cup of water. Preparation Technique: Place the blueberries, radishes, and water in a blender. Blend until smooth. Serve the mixture after straining it through a sieve.

8. Plum Tomato Juice - Ingredients: 4 plums, 4 tomatoes, 1 cup of water. Preparation Technique: Peel and chop the plums. Peel and chop the tomatoes. Place the chopped plums, chopped tomatoes, and water in a blender. Blend until smooth. Serve the mixture after straining it through a sieve.

9. Grape Kale Juice - Ingredients: 1 cup grapes, 2 cups kale leaves, 1 cup of water. Preparation Technique: Place the grapes, kale leaves, and water in a blender. Blend until smooth. Serve the mixture after straining it through a sieve.

10. Orange Coconut Juice - Ingredients: 2 oranges, 1 cup coconut milk, 1 cup of water. Preparation Technique: Peel and chop the oranges. Place the chopped oranges, coconut milk, and water in a blender. Blend until smooth. Serve the mixture after straining it through a sieve.

11. Mango Parsley Juice - Ingredients: 2 mangos, 1 cup parsley leaves, 1 cup of water. Preparation Technique: Peel and chop the mangos. Place the chopped mangos, parsley leaves, and water in a blender. Blend until smooth. Serve the mixture after straining it through a sieve.

12. Cantaloupe Mint Juice - Ingredients: 1 cantaloupe, 1 cup mint leaves, 1 cup of water. Preparation Technique: Peel and chop the cantaloupe. Place the chopped cantaloupe, mint leaves, and water in a blender. Blend until smooth. Serve the mixture after straining it through a sieve.

13. Apple Celery Juice - Ingredients: 2 apples, 2 stalks celery, 1 cup of water. Preparation Technique: Peel and chop the apples. Place the chopped apples, celery, and water in a blender. Blend until smooth. Serve the mixture after straining it through a sieve.

14. Watermelon Lettuce Juice - Ingredients: 1 cup watermelon, 2 cups lettuce leaves, 1 cup of water. Preparation Technique: Peel

and chop the watermelon. Place the chopped watermelon, lettuce leaves, and water in a blender. Blend until smooth. Serve the mixture after straining it through a sieve.

15. Pineapple Beet Juice - Ingredients: 1 cup pineapple, 1 beet, 1 cup of water. Preparation Technique: Peel and chop the pineapple. Peel and grate the beet. Place the chopped pineapple, grated beet, and water in a blender. Blend until smooth. Serve the mixture after straining it through a sieve.

16. Peach Broccoli Juice - Ingredients: 2 peaches, 2 cups broccoli florets, 1 cup of water. Preparation Technique: Peel and chop the peaches. Place the chopped peaches, broccoli florets, and water in a blender. Blend until smooth. Serve the mixture after straining it through a sieve.

17. Carrot Tomato Juice - Ingredients: 3 carrots, 4 tomatoes, 1 cup of water. Preparation Technique: Peel and chop the carrots. Peel and chop the tomatoes. Place the chopped carrots, chopped tomatoes, and water in a blender. Blend until smooth. Serve the mixture after straining it through a sieve.

18. Kiwi Spinach Juice - Ingredients: 2 kiwis, 2 cups spinach leaves, 1 cup of water. Preparation Technique: Peel and chop the kiwis. Place the chopped kiwis, spinach leaves, and water in a blender. Blend until smooth. Serve the mixture after straining it through a sieve.

19. Lemon Parsley Juice - Ingredients: 2 lemons, 1 cup parsley leaves, 1 cup of water. Preparation Technique: Peel and chop the lemons. Place the chopped lemons, parsley leaves, and water in a blender. Blend until smooth. Serve the mixture after straining it through a sieve.

20. Avocado Kale Juice - Ingredients: 1 avocado, 2 cups kale leaves, 1 cup of water. Preparation Technique: Peel and pit the avocado. Place the avocado, kale leaves, and water in a blender. Blend until smooth. Serve the mixture after straining it through a sieve.

21. Coconut Radish Juice - Ingredients: 1 cup coconut milk, 2 radishes, 1 cup of water. Preparation Technique: Place the coconut milk, radishes, and water in a blender. Blend until smooth. Serve the mixture after straining it through a sieve.

22. Blueberry Mint Juice - Ingredients: 1 cup blueberries, 1 cup mint leaves, 1 cup of water. Preparation Technique: Place the blueberries, mint leaves, and water in a blender. Blend until smooth. Serve the mixture after straining it through a sieve.

23. Plum Celery Juice - Ingredients: 4 plums, 2 stalks celery, 1 cup of water. Preparation Technique: Peel and chop the plums. Place the chopped plums, celery, and water in a blender. Blend until smooth. Serve the mixture after straining it through a sieve.

24. Grape Coconut Juice - Ingredients: 1 cup grapes, 1 cup coconut milk, 1 cup of water. Preparation Technique: Place the grapes, coconut milk, and water in a blender. Blend until smooth. Serve the mixture after straining it through a sieve.

25. Orange Lettuce Juice - Ingredients: 2 oranges, 2 cups lettuce leaves, 1 cup of water. Preparation Technique: Peel and chop the oranges. Place the chopped oranges, lettuce leaves, and water in a blender. Blend until smooth. Serve the mixture after straining it through a sieve.

IMPORTANCE OF BALANCING SWEET AND TART FLAVORS IN JUICING RECIPES

Balancing sweet and tart flavors in juicing recipes is important because it creates a more enjoyable taste experience for the drinker. Too much sweetness can be overwhelming and lead to a sugar crash, while too much tartness can be unpleasantly sour. By balancing the sweet and tart flavors, you can create a harmonious blend of flavors that is both refreshing and satisfying.

When it comes to choosing the best citrus fruits for juicing, there are a few key factors to consider:

Juice yield:

Some citrus fruits, like lemons and limes, are very juicy and yield a lot of juice per fruit, while others, like grapefruits, may yield less juice. Consider the juice yield of the fruit when choosing which ones to juice.

Sweetness vs. tartness:

Different citrus fruits have varying levels of sweetness and tartness. For example, oranges are generally sweeter than lemons.

When choosing citrus fruits for juicing, consider the balance of sweet and tart flavors you want to achieve in your juice.

Seasonality:

Citrus fruits are often at their best during the winter months, but some varieties may be available year-round. Choosing seasonal fruits can ensure that you are getting the freshest, most flavorful fruits.

TIPS FOR CHOOSING THE BEST CITRUS FRUITS FOR JUICING

Choose ripe fruits:

Ripe citrus fruits will be juicier and more flavorful than unripe ones. Look for fruits that are heavy for their size and have a slight give when squeezed.

Mix and match:

Experiment with different combinations of citrus fruits to achieve the flavor profile you want. For example, mixing sweet oranges with tart lemons can create a balanced, refreshing juice.

Use a citrus press or juicer:

Using a citrus press or juicer can help you extract the maximum amount of juice from your citrus fruits. This can be especially helpful if you are juicing a large quantity of fruits.

By balancing sweet and tart flavors in your juicing recipes and choosing the best citrus fruits, you can create delicious and refreshing juices that are both healthy and enjoyable.

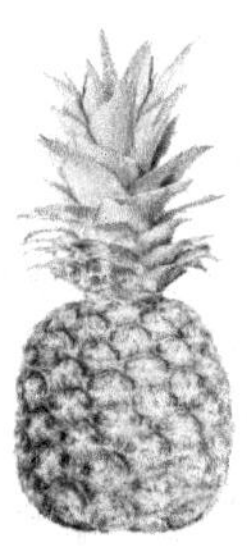

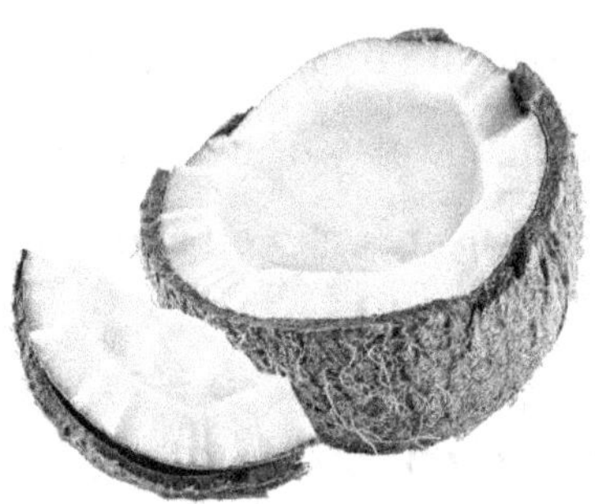

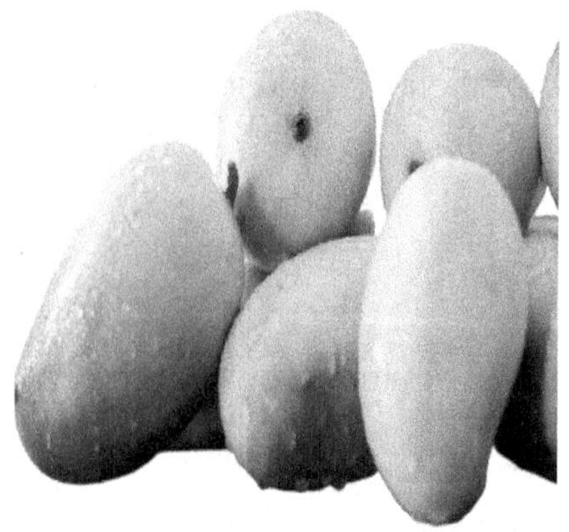

CHAPTER 4

TIPS FOR JUICING WITH DIABETES

USE FRESH PRODUCE :

Using fresh produce for juicing with diabetes is an excellent idea. Fresh produce contains more vitamins and minerals than processed produce and can help to regulate blood sugar levels. Fresh fruits and vegetables are also full of antioxidants, fiber, and other important nutrients that can help manage diabetes. Additionally, fresh produce is often higher in fiber and lower in sugar than processed produce, making it a healthier choice for those with diabetes. When juicing with diabetes, it is important to choose fruits and vegetables that are low in sugar and high in fiber. Choosing seasonal produce is a great way to ensure that you are getting the freshest and most nutritious ingredients. Additionally, adding fresh herbs and spices to your juice can add flavor and additional health benefits. Juicing can be a great way to manage diabetes and get a healthy dose of nutrients. By using fresh produce and adding healthy ingredients to your juice, you can enjoy delicious and nutritious juice while helping to manage your diabetes.

MONITOR BLOOD GLUCOSE LEVEL:

Juicing with diabetes can be a great way to get natural vitamins, minerals, and fiber into your diet. It is important to remember, however, that many fruit and vegetable juices can contain high levels of sugar and carbohydrates, which can affect your blood glucose levels. To ensure that you are juicing safely, it is important to monitor your blood glucose levels before, during, and after juicing.

Before you start juicing, check your blood glucose level to make sure it is within a safe range. If it is too high or too low, it is best to wait until it is in a safe range before juicing.

During juicing, you should monitor your blood glucose levels every 30 minutes or so. This will help you gauge how your body is responding to the juice and what adjustments you may need to make.

Finally, after you have finished juicing, check your blood glucose levels again. If your blood glucose levels have increased significantly, you may need to adjust your diet and exercise routine to ensure that your blood glucose remains in a safe range.

By monitoring your blood glucose levels before, during, and after juicing, you can ensure that you are juicing safely with diabetes.

LISTEN TO YOUR BODY

Listening to your body is a key tip for juicing with diabetes. When you listen to your body, you can make sure you are consuming the right amount of nutrients, vitamins, and fiber to help manage your diabetes. You can also pay attention to any side effects that may be associated with certain juices. For example, some juices may contain a high amount of sugar, so it is important to pay attention to how much sugar is in the juice and how it affects your blood sugar levels. Additionally, certain juices may also trigger an allergy or other food sensitivity, so it is important to understand how your body responds to different ingredients. Finally, listening to your body can provide invaluable information regarding how certain juices make you feel. If you feel energized and satisfied after drinking a certain juice, then you can be sure to include it in your diet. However, if you feel sluggish or nauseous after drinking a particular juice, then it is best to avoid it. Listening to your body is an important tip for juicing with diabetes as it can help you create a healthy and balanced diet.

CONSIDER NUTRIENT CONTENT

When it comes to juicing with diabetes, considering nutrient content is an important tip. Nutrients are essential for managing diabetes, so it's important to be aware of which fruits and vegetables are high in beneficial nutrients.

Fruits and vegetables that are high in fiber, vitamins, and minerals are typically the best choices. Examples include apples, carrots, spinach, kale, blueberries, oranges, and grapefruit. These fruits and vegetables are packed with vitamins, minerals, and fiber, which help to keep blood sugar in check. Additionally, they contain antioxidants that help to reduce inflammation and protect cells from damage.

When juicing, it's important to use a variety of fruits and vegetables to ensure that you are getting a wide range of beneficial nutrients. Additionally, avoid adding sugar or artificial sweeteners to the juices. These can quickly increase blood sugar levels, which can be dangerous for those with diabetes.

Finally, be sure to monitor your blood sugar levels before and after juicing. This will help to ensure that the juices are not causing an unexpected spike in blood sugar levels. With some careful planning and consideration of nutrient content, juicing can be a healthy and delicious way to manage diabetes.

CHOOSE LOW GLYCEMIC FRUITS AND VEGETABLES: Juicing with diabetes can be a tricky endeavor, and it's important to be mindful of the glycemic index of the fruits and vegetables you're using. Low-glycemic fruits and vegetables are the best choice for people with diabetes, as they have a less dramatic effect on blood sugar levels. The glycemic index is a measure of how quickly a particular food affects blood sugar levels, and low-glycemic foods have a score lower than 55.

When choosing fruits and vegetables for juicing, look for those with a low glycemic index. Apples, pears, strawberries, oranges, grapefruit, peaches, blueberries, and raspberries are all great choices. You may also want to consider adding some vegetables, such as kale, cucumbers, celery, spinach, and peppers. Additionally, adding some low-glycemic nuts, such as almonds and walnuts, can give your juice an extra boost of nutrition.

When juicing with diabetes, it's important to keep track of the amount of carbohydrates you're consuming. Be sure to measure the fruits and vegetables you're using, and don't forget to include the carbohydrates from any added nuts or seeds. Additionally, it's important to limit the amount of added sugar in your juice. If you need to sweeten your juice, try adding some stevia or honey.

By choosing low-glycemic fruits and vegetables, as well as limiting added sugar, you can safely enjoy a cup of freshly-squeezed juice while managing your diabetes.

AVOID HIGH SUGAR JUICES

When it comes to juicing with diabetes, avoiding high sugar juices is paramount. High sugar juices can cause your blood sugar to rapidly spike, which can be dangerous for those with diabetes. To avoid this, choose fruits and vegetables that are low in sugar such as cucumber, celery, kale, and spinach. Additionally, you can add some tart fruits such as grapefruit, lemon, and lime to add flavor without the added sugar. Also, consider adding herbs and spices like ginger and garlic to your juice for flavor and health benefits. Finally, if you do choose higher sugar fruits like apples and oranges, be sure to use them in moderation. By following these tips, you can enjoy the benefits of juicing while managing your diabetes.

BALANCE JIUCE WITH WHOLE FOODS

Balancing juice with whole foods is a great tip for juicing with diabetes. Juicing is a great way to get a wide variety of vitamins, minerals, and antioxidants into your diet, but it's important to think about how to balance these juices with other healthy whole foods. Eating whole foods can help keep your blood sugar levels in check, while also providing more fiber and other essential nutrients. When juicing, focus on adding some whole fruits and vegetables to your juice, such as apples, carrots, kale, and spinach. These will help provide additional fiber and other essential vitamins and minerals that are not found in juice. Additionally, try to minimize added sugars and sweeteners, as these can contribute to a rise in blood sugar levels. Finally, be sure to drink plenty of water throughout the day to help keep your body hydrated and flush out toxins. By following these tips, you can enjoy the benefits of juicing while helping to keep your diabetes under control.

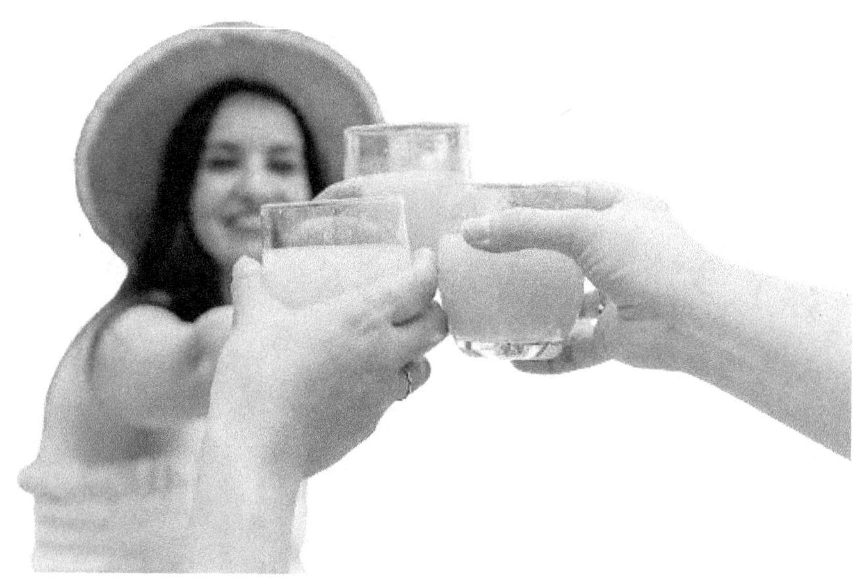

CONCLUSION

Juicing has a number of potential benefits for those with diabetes. It can help regulate blood glucose levels, reduce inflammation, and provide essential vitamins and minerals. Additionally, juicing can help to reduce overall calorie intake and encourage healthier dietary choices. Finally, juicing can provide an opportunity to add in beneficial foods such as leafy greens, celery, and ginger, which can help to reduce the risk of complications associated with diabetes. In summary, juicing can be a great way to support a healthy diet and lifestyle for those with diabetes.

Consulting with a healthcare professional can help individuals with diabetes determine whether juicing is a good choice for them and how to incorporate it safely into their diet.

A healthcare professional, such as a registered dietitian or a certified diabetes educator, can help individuals with diabetes create a well-balanced, nutritious diet that meets their unique needs. They can also provide guidance on how to safely incorporate juicing into their dietary plan while managing their blood sugar levels.

Moreover, healthcare professionals can provide insight on the potential risks of juicing, such as high sugar and carbohydrate content, and how to choose the right fruits and vegetables to juice for individuals with diabetes.

In conclusion, it is always advisable to seek the advice of a healthcare professional before making significant changes to your diet, especially if you have diabetes. Consulting with a healthcare professional can help individuals with diabetes make informed decisions about their dietary choices and improve their overall health and wellbeing.

www.ingramcontent.com/pod-product-compliance
Lightning Source LLC
Chambersburg PA
CBHW061556250726
48657CB00021B/1913